Raw Cannabis:
Juicing Fresh Cannabis Leaf

The Medicinal Benefits of Cannabis

By Ryder Management Inc.

PROLOGUE

"Let food be thy medicine and medicine be thy food."
Hippocrates

"In the absence of the sacred, nothing is sacred – everything is for sale"
Oren Lyons, Onondaga, 1992

.

Table of Contents

Overview

The effectiveness of cannabis has typically been reported according to its THC content, the psychoactive effectiveness. THC is obtained from the cannabinoid THC acid (Tetrahydrocannabinolic Acid or THCA) through the process of decarboxylation or heating. This process is also known as activating the cannabinoid. THC can also be derived through aging. To think of cannabis according only to its psychotropic ability restricts or otherwise prevents the number of other health and medicinal benefits that can be derived from this plant.

Cannabis, in its raw or unheated form, provides a plethora of essential nutrients and benefits, none of which have psychotropic effects. Dr. William Courtney refers to cannabis in its raw form as a daily essential and classifies it as a vegetable. In addition to the many benefits of cannabinoids in their raw form (cannabinoid acids), cannabis also produces many beneficial terpenes. When terpenes are chemically modified such as by oxidation (curing or drying), they are then referred to as terpenoids. Therefore, by consuming cannabis in its raw form, one benefits from both its cannabinoids and terpenes and the synergistic effect is nothing short of amazing as the plant contains a multitude of medicinal and health benefits, as a whole.

In order to provide an understanding of the huge benefits that cannabis offers in its raw form, it is important to know the science behind this plant. This book includes an in-depth look at cannabinoid acids and some of the more common terpenes found in cannabis. Additionally, tips and suggestions on juicing cannabis are also provided to assist in the consumption of cannabis in its raw form. Also included are the benefits of consuming hemp seed including hemp seed oil, another important super food that was previously denied to the masses.

Recent studies reveal that cannabinoid acids possess both analgesic and anti -inflammatory properties. For this and other reasons, this book is focused on cannabis in its raw form.

Cannabinoids

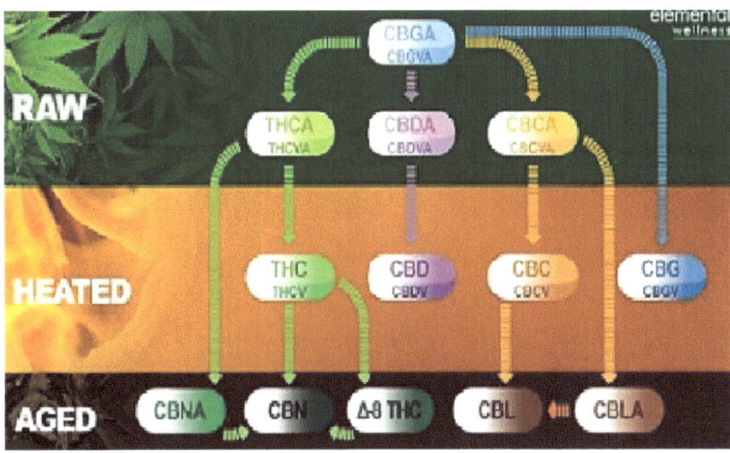

Cannabinoids have been defined as plant secondary metabolites which mean that as organic compounds, they are not directly involved in the normal growth, development or reproduction of the plant. However, secondary plant metabolites, although not yet fully understood by the scientific community, are important for a plant (and humans) to thrive. Scientists are now drawing the conclusion that the primary purpose of phyto-cannabinoids, cannabinoids found in plants, are to enhance and regulate our endocannabinoid system.

Phyto-cannabinoids begin by possessing either olivetol or olivetolic acid. The cannabinoid acids also possess monoterpene groups in their molecules. Monoterpenes prevent the carcinogenesis process at both the initiation and promotion/ progression stages of cancer and have been found to be effective in treating early and advanced cancers. There have been a number of cannabinoids isolated from the cannabis plant including from her fresh fan leaves.

Although there have been approximately eighty cannabinoids identified, it is believed that all cannabinoids are derived from Cannabigerolic Acid or CBGA. The above picture, from Elemental Wellness, illustrates the origin of the various cannabinoids and how they can exist in various forms depending on whether they have been heated or not.

The ability of the cannabis plant to produce Cannabigerolic Acid (CBGA) is what makes this plant so unique. Cannabigerolic Acid, as illustrated in the above picture from Elemental Wellness, is the precursor to the three main branches of cannabinoid acids: Tetrahydrocannabinolic Acid (THCA, Cannabidiolic Acid (CBDA) and Cannabichromenic Acid (CBCA).

Cannabis preparation techniques are based on the benefits desired from the plant, as the plant is able to treat and cure a myriad of symptoms and diseases. By juicing the cannabis plant, one is able to receive the most beneficial medical benefits from this special plant without the "high" associated with the THC. Dr. William Courtney believes that cannabis, in its raw form, is one of the best preventive medicines known and also believes that cannabis is one of the most important vegetable on the planet and should be treated and thought of as a dietary essential.

It is also important to remember that terpenes remain intact when consuming fresh cannabis and this plant in its raw form has no psycho active ability.

The following pages describe the major cannabinoid acids and their benefits followed by a description of the more commonly found terpenes along with their benefits.

Cannabigerolic Acid (CBGA)

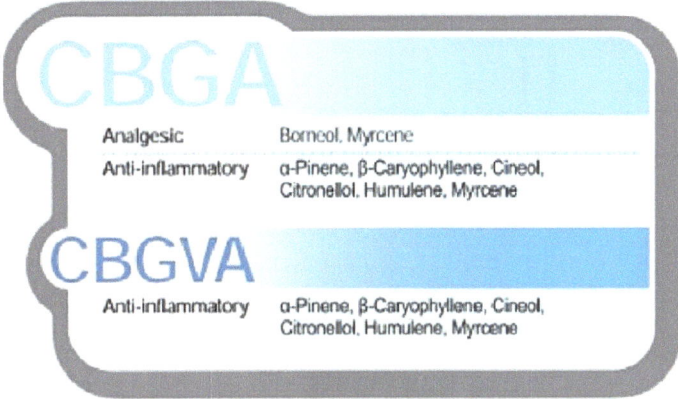

Formula: C22 H31 O4

The above illustration discloses, on the right, the terpenes associated with each noted acidic cannabinoid.

Cannabigerolic acid or CBGA is probably the most important factor in creating the health benefits associated with cannabis. Cannabigerolic Acid is said to possess all the health benefits associated with medical cannabis. It is primarily known for reducing inflammation, pain relief and it has been shown to slow bacterial growth.

Cannabigerolic acid is formed from a combination of Geraryl pyrophosphate and olivetolic acid.

Pharmacological characteristics of CBGA, according to Bloom Well, is Antibiotic

Cannabidiolic Acid (CBDA)

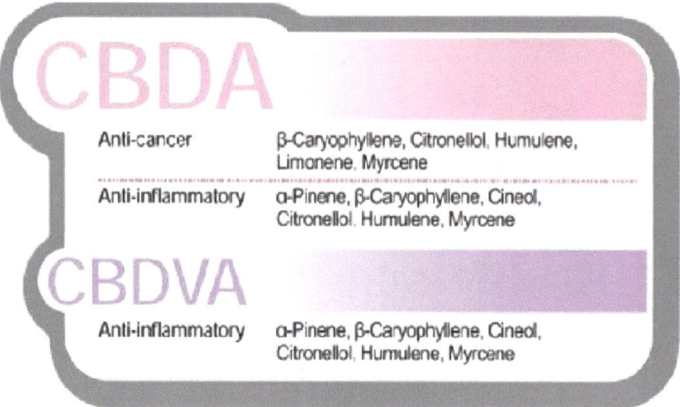

Formula: C22 H30 O4
Decarboxylation temperature: 120 + C (248 F)

Cannabidiolic Acid or CBDA was previously found mainly in Ruderalis or hemp species of cannabis. It is one of the four possible outcomes of Cannabigerolic acid. The US patent 6,630,507 B1 dated October 7, 2003 reports that CBDA is more potent than either Vitamin C or Vitamin E in their functions.

CBDA reduces inflammation and inhibits cancer cell growth. As the precursor to CBD, it seems logical to conclude that CBDA also contains the astounding benefits associated with CBD, CBDA in its activated form.

Tetrahydrocannabinolic Acid (THCA)

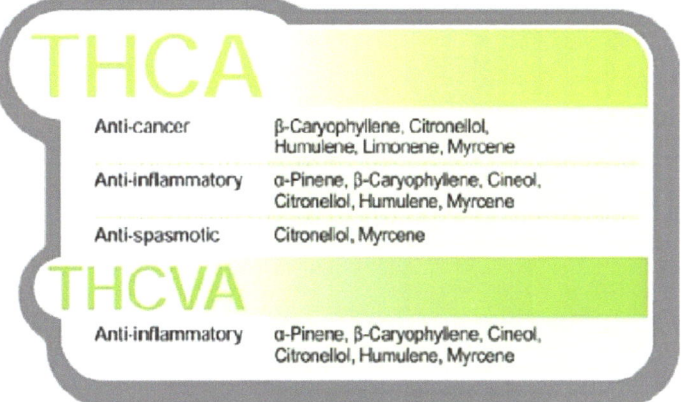

THCA	
Anti-cancer	β-Caryophyllene, Citronellol, Humulene, Limonene, Myrcene
Anti-inflammatory	α-Pinene, β-Caryophyllene, Cineol, Citronellol, Humulene, Myrcene
Anti-spasmotic	Citronellol, Myrcene
THCVA	
Anti-inflammatory	α-Pinene, β-Caryophyllene, Cineol, Citronellol, Humulene, Myrcene

Formula: C22 H30 O4
Boiling Point: 105C (220 F)

As with other cannabinoid acids, THC-A is non-psychoactive. THC-A has many medicinal and health benefits including anti-inflammatory, anti-tumor, its ability to fight insomnia, and is anti-spasmodic effectiveness.

It is interesting to note that US patent number 7,807,711 B2 is a patent on using a combination of mainly THCA with CBDA and CBGA for relieving pain, suppressing an inflammatory response, and for treating certain diseases including autoimmune and inflammatory diseases including treating the symptoms associated with those conditions.

Cannabichromic Acid (CBCA)

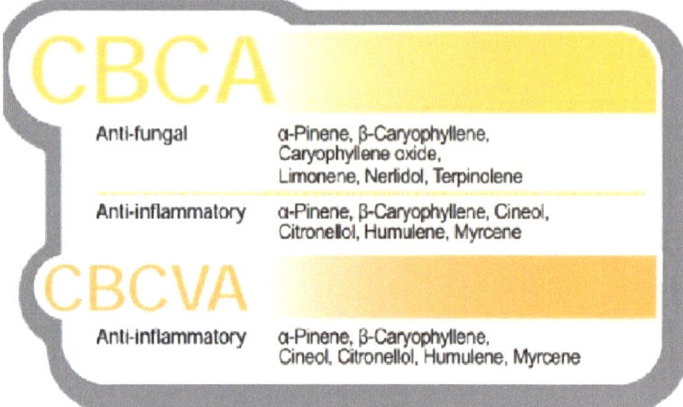

CBCA	
Anti-fungal	α-Pinene, β-Caryophyllene, Caryophyllene oxide, Limonene, Nerlidol, Terpinolene
Anti-inflammatory	α-Pinene, β-Caryophyllene, Cineol, Citronellol, Humulene, Myrcene
CBCVA	
Anti-inflammatory	α-Pinene, β-Caryophyllene, Cineol, Citronellol, Humulene, Myrcene

Formula: C22 H30 O4

Cannabichromic acid or CBCA is the third major branch of cannabinoids from CBGA. A recent patent claims that CBCA is produced primarily in the sessile trichomes of the plant (those without stock). CBCA contains anti -inflammatory, antifungal and antibacterial properties. This makes CBCA an effective treatment for fungal infections and the reduction of inflammation in the body.

Cannabicyclol Acid (CBLA)

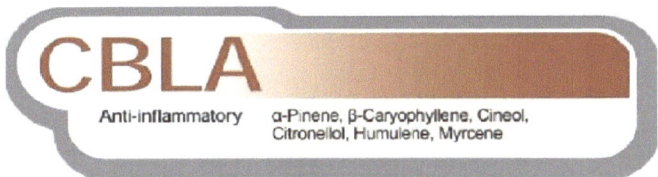

Formula: C22 H30 O4

Cannabicyclol acid or CBLA is a degradation product. When CBCA absorbs UV light, CBLA is produced.

This is not to say that degradation means inactive, CBLA still contains anti-inflammatory properties.

Cannabinolic Acid (CBNA)

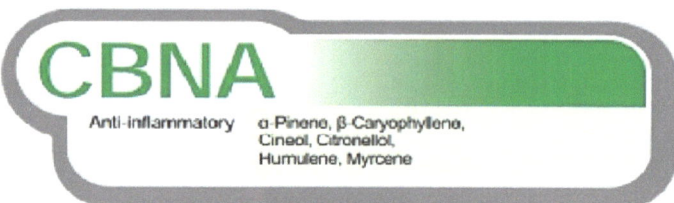

Formula: *C28 H42 O4*

Cannabinolic acid or CBNA is a breakdown product of THCA by air oxidation.

The Importance of Terpenes

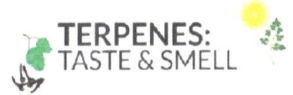

Terpenes are a large and diverse class of naturally occurring organic compounds produced by a number of plants of which many are "aromatic hydrocarbons" (sometimes called arenes). When terpenes are chemically modified such as by oxidation, they are referred to as terpenoids. Terpenoids are also known as isoprenoids. Terpenes and terpenoids are the primary constituents of the essential oils of many plants and flowers including cannabis. The difference between terpenes and terpenoids is that terpenes are hydrocarbons whereas terpenoids contain "additional functional groups" (meaning they contain specific groups of atoms). Terpenes are volatile which means they can easily evaporate at normal temperatures or are liable to change quite rapidly and unpredictably, sometimes for the worse. They are the compounds in cannabis, as with other plants, that give rise to the plant's unique scent. Since cannabinoids have no smell, the unique scent within a cannabis strain is due to a unique combination of its terpenes.

Terpenes are more volatile than cannabinoids and their presence relates to the freshness of the strain. It has long been known that therapeutic benefits can be had through aromatherapy, a form of alternative medicine that uses volatile plant materials and other aromatic compounds for health and other beneficial purposes. Therefore, just like the cannabinoids in cannabis, the terpenes in cannabis also produce many health benefits.

Terpenes are referred to as terpenoids when they are denatured by oxidation such as when the cannabis plant has been dried and cured. Terpenes are also considered terpenoids when they have been chemically altered by some rearrangement of the carbon skeleton.

There are approximately 120 known and distinct terpenes produced by the cannabis plant and the relative concentration of the individual terpenes varies considerably among the different strains of cannabis. Laboratory experiments have shown that it is impossible to recreate Cannabis resin to include the full medicinal effect that the cannabis plant is able to offer, by simply synthesizing some of the cannabinoids contained within cannabis.

From a chemical standpoint, terpenes are a large and varied class of hydrocarbons that make up a majority of plant resins and sap. The name terpene comes from "turpentine", which, in its raw form, is the sap from the Pine tree and which is terpene based. Essential oils are primarily composed of terpenes and have a very long history of use in medicine both topically and internally

Terpenes are derived biosynthetically from units of isoprene (a colorless volatile liquid produced by many plants) with the molecular formula *C5H8*. The basic molecular formulae for terpenes are multiples of this basic formula or *(C5H8) n, where "n" is the number of isoprene units.* This is known as the C5 rule. The isoprene units can link "head to tail" to form linear chains or they can arrange themselves to form rings. An isoprene unit is considered one of Nature's common building blocks.

As isoprene units join together, the resulting terpenes are then classified according to sequential size. For example, a prefix to the terpene name is added to indicate the number of terpene units necessary to make up the molecule:

*Hemi*terpenes: a single isoprene unit

*Mono*terpenes: two isoprene units with the molecular formula C10H16

*Sesqui*terpenes: three isoprene units with the molecular formula C15H24

Bicyclic terpenes feature two fused rings.

Monoterpenes and sesquiterpenes are found to make up

approximately 90% of the terpenes found in the cannabis plant.

Pinene

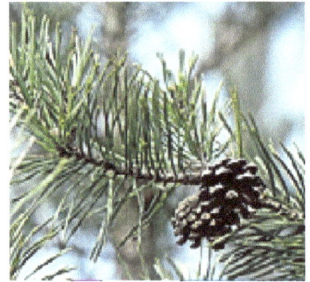

Formula: C10H16
Boiling Point: 155C (311 F)

In addition to the cannabis plant, Pinene can be found in abundance in Pine Trees and is one of the major constituents of terpenic oil, which has been used in healing for centuries. There are two structural isomers of pinene found in nature: alpha or a-pinene and beta or b-pinene. Pinene is important physiologically in not only both plants and animals, but also in our environment. A-Pinene reacts with a number of other chemicals and then forms other terpenes such as delta-Limonene (D-Limonene).

Alpha-Pinene is anti-inflammatory and has been used for centuries as a bronchodilator in the treatment of asthma and cystic fibrosis. Other medicinal benefits of this terpene include: anti-bacterial, anti-fungal, anti-inflammatory, and expectorant and it has been found to increase mental focus and alertness.

A-Pinene can also be found in orange peels and other citrus rinds and in the medicinal essential oils of rosemary, basil, parsley, dill along with the eucalyptus tree.

Beta-Caryophyllene (BCP)

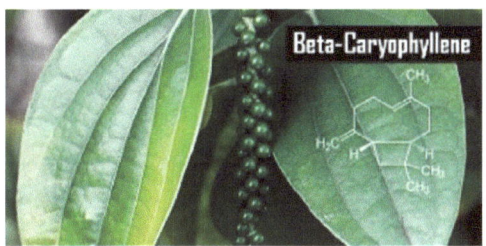

Formula: C15H24
Boiling Point: 160C (320 F)

Beta-caryophyllene, a *bicyclic sesquiterpene*, is found in many plants, in addition to cannabis. These plants include Thai basils; cloves; hops; along with oregano, rosemary, cinnamon bark and black pepper. The aroma is therefore said to be spicy, peppery and/or woody.

Sesquiterpenes are a class of terpenes that consist of three isoprene units rather than two such as that found in monoterpenes.

Research has shown that B-Caryophyllene has a natural attraction to the CB2 endocannabinoid receptor found in the human body. Beta-caryophyllene is known to be antiseptic, antifungal, anti-inflammatory, antibacterial, antitumor, bronchodilator and is found to also be effective at reducing neuropathic pain. This terpene also has gastro-protective qualities and is good for gastrointestinal complications. BCP also binds to the CB2 receptor, in fact, it acts specifically on the body's CB2 cannabinoid pathways and since CB2 is considered an endocannabinoid receptor (found in the body) BCP is also being considered a cannabinoid.

It is this scent that trainers teach drug dogs to find. This terpene also has gastro-protective qualities and is good for gastrointestinal complications. BCP also binds to the CB2 receptor, in fact, it acts specifically on the body's CB2 cannabinoid pathways and since CB2 is considered an endocannabinoid receptor (found in the body) BCP is being considered a cannabinoid. It is this scent that trainers teach drug dogs to find. Cannabis strains known to contain a high content of BCP include the Indica Hash Plant. Cannabis strains known to contain a high content of BCP include the Indica Hash Plant.

Cineole

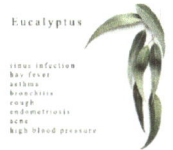

Formula: C10 H18 O
Boiling point: 177C (450 F)

Cineol, also known as eucalyptol, is found in many plants including bay leaf, tea tree, mugwort, sweet basil, wormwood, rosemary, common sage in addition to cannabis. Cineol is insoluble in water but miscible with ether, ethanol or chloroform.

Therapeutic benefits include pain relief, increased circulation, anti-bacterial, anti-depressant, anti-inflammatory and bronchodilator.

Cineole is variable across the various cannabis strains but has been found as a major component of the essential oil.

Eucalyptus and the cineole chemotype of rosemary are on the list of essential oils to avoid using on children under the age of ten years.

Citronellol

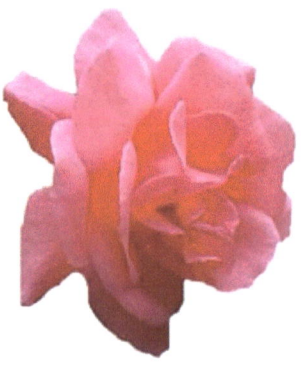

Formula: C10 H20 O
Boiling Point: 225C (437 F)

Citronellol is a monoterpene that is used in perfumes and insect repellents. Citronellol is also an effective mosquito repellent at short distances.

As a medicinal compound, this terpene is found to be helpful as a sleep aid and it also contains anti-tumor, anti-inflammatory and antispasmodic properties.

Citronellol is found in abundance in many varieties of roses.

Humulene

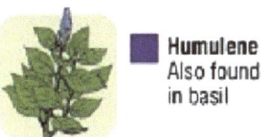

Humulene
Also found
in basil

Anti-inflamatory

Robust
Herbaceous
Earth

Formula: C15H24
Boiling Point: 198C (388 F)

Humulene is a sesquiterpene and has the same formula as Beta-caryophyllene. Humulene is found in hops and Vietnamese coriander, in addition to various strains of cannabis and other plants. This terpene is anorectic meaning that it suppresses appetite. It is also anti-tumor, anti-bacterial and anti-inflammatory. In Traditional Chinese Medicine (TCM), Humulene is commonly combined with beta-caryophyllene and used as an effective remedy for inflammation.

Limonene

Limonene Also found in citrus	Treats acid reflux Anti-anxiety Antidepressant	Citrus Fresh spice

Formula: C10 H16
Boiling Point: 176C (349 F)

Limonene has a strong citrus odor and bitter taste and is useful in treating depression and anxiety. Limonene has the ability to permeate proteins thus making it effective in the treatment of toenail fungus. It is also found to be anti-cancerous in parallel with boosting the immune system. Limonene is also one of the two major compounds formed from alpha-Pinene. As a major aromatic compound in essential oils, limonene's potential effects on cellular metabolism have been elusive when studied.

Limonene is found in cannabis resin and tropical fruit rinds.

Limonene is an anti-bacterial, anti-fungal and anti-cancer agent. Limonene is also able to increase the absorption of other terpenes by making cell membranes more permeable.

Linalool

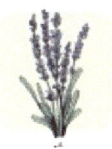

Linalool
Also found
in lavender

Anesthetic
Anti-convulsive
Analgesic
Anti-anxiety

Flowers
Lavender
Citrus
Fresh spice

Formula: C10 H1 O
Boiling Point 198C (388 F)

Linalool is a simple terpene alcohol and has been found in over 200 plant species including lavenders, citrus, laurels, birch, coriander and rosewood. This terpene has been used for thousands of years as a sleep aid. Linalool is also a very important precursor in the formation of Vitamin E. Linalool also has anti-anxiety properties and therefore has been used in the treatment of both psychosis and anxiety disorders and has also been used as an anti-epileptic agent. Linalool has also been used to treat depression and for pain relief. The vapors of linalool have been found to be effective against fruit flies, fleas and cockroaches.

Myrcene

Myrcene	Sedative	Flowers
Also found	Sleep aid	Pungent
in hops	Muscle relaxant	Earth

Formula: C10H16
Boiling Point: 168C (334 F)

Myrcene is a very important monoterpene as it is a precursor in the formation of other terpenes. Beta-Myrcene can also be found in mango, bay leaves, eucalyptus, lemongrass and more. B-Myrcene is effective in providing pain relief and is also anti-tumor and anti-inflammatory. It is also known to be effective in treating insomnia and is also used in the treatment of spasms. Beta-Myrcene also is able to lower the resistance across the blood to brain barrier facilitating it and other chemicals to cross the barrier. What this means in the case of THC is that it allows it to take effect more quickly. It has also been shown that this terpene increases the maximum saturation level of the CB1 receptor, improving the uptake of many beneficial chemical compounds.

Terpinolene

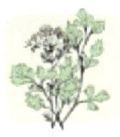

Terpinolene Analgesic Pine
Also found Pain reduction Herbal
in coriander Digestive aid Anise
  Stomachic Lime

Formula: C10H16
Boiling Point: 174C

Terpinolene is from a group of terpenes called *terpinenes*. This group of isomeric hydrocarbons each has the same molecular formula and carbon framework, but they differ in the position of the carbon-carbon double bonds.

δ-Terpinene, also known as Terpinolene, is found in abundance in coriander (also known as cilantro) along with apples, cumin, lilac, tea tree and many conifers. The scent is a soft woody smoke. Terpinolene has been used as an anti-septic for centuries and it also contains anti-bacterial and anti-fungal properties.

Cannabis Synergy

In his paper *"Taming THC: potential cannabis synergy and phytocannabinoid-terpenoid entourage effects"* published in the August, 2011 **British Journal of Pharmacology**, Ethan Russo, a scientist with GW Pharmaceuticals, wrote "cannabis has been a medicinal plant of unparalleled versatility for millennia but whose mechanisms of action were an unsolved mystery .." until the following three discoveries: THC, CB1 - the first discovered cannabinoid receptor and the endocannabinoid system.

After identifying the specific terpenes found in cannabis, Russo mentions the potential synergistic medicinal benefits of the terpenes and terpenoids to the cannabinoids and states that the identified terpenes in cannabis have individually been designated as "Generally Recognized as Safe" by the US FDA and other regulatory agencies, prior to his following written summary on this subject:

"They display unique therapeutic effects that may contribute meaningfully to the entourage effects of cannabis-based medicinal extracts. Particular focus will be placed on phytocannabinoid-terpenoid interactions that could produce synergy with respect to treatment of pain, inflammation, depression, anxiety, addiction, epilepsy, cancer, fungal and bacterial infections (including methicillin-resistant Staphylococcus aureus). Scientific evidence is presented for non-cannabinoid plant components as putative antidotes to intoxicating effects of THC that could increase its therapeutic index. Methods for investigating entourage effects in future experiments will be proposed. Phytocannabinoid-terpenoid synergy, if proven, increases the likelihood that an extensive pipeline of new therapeutic products is possible from this venerable plant."

Although the scientific study is exciting in terms of providing further scientific proof on the medical benefits of cannabis, proof that previously was said to be lacking, it should be noted that GW Pharmaceuticals have a number of patents and patent applications regarding the medicinal use of cannabis in numerous methods of delivery.

The report does describe the importance of the fan leaves in terms of the creation of cannabinoids and terpenes in "secretory cells inside glandular trichomes", the potential ability of the fan leaves to assist in one's health care should not be overlooked.

Tips and Suggestions on Juicing Cannabis

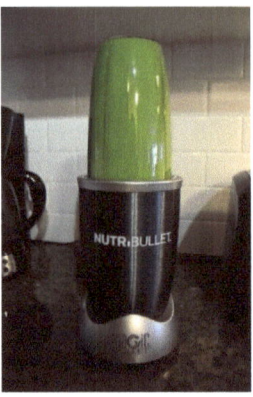

Dr. William Courtney recommends that patient's juice eight to fifteen leaves a day. This can be simply and easily prepared by using a blender along with one or two cups of filtered or distilled water.

In order to reap all the benefits, it is recommended not to strain the juiced cannabis because the cannabis fiber contains important fiber content. David Wolfe's "NutriBullet" is ideal for juicing cannabis.

When it comes to juicing, as with any vegetable, the fresher the product, the better.

If you find that the taste of raw cannabis juice is a little bitter, mixing it with another vegetable or fruit juice will help. Cannabis that has been cured or dried and prepared for smoking is not suitable for juicing.

Split your drink into three parts for consumption at each meal.

As you pick a plant, also plant a plant in order to have a continuous supply of fresh cannabis to juice.

Raw cannabis, not rinsed, can be stored in the refrigerator in freezer bags that extend the freshness of vegetables.

Raw bud has the highest concentration of cannabinoids, more so than the leaves, and is an excellent source for consumption if resources allow this.

Some say that the leaves for eating or juicing should be picked from plants that are well into their flowering stage for maximum benefits. However, fan leaves also provide a plethora of health benefits alone.

As with any vegetable used for consumption, using a diluted spray of Food Grade Hydrogen Peroxide (FGHP) is the safest and best method of ensuring the least amount of contaminants.

Hemp Benefits

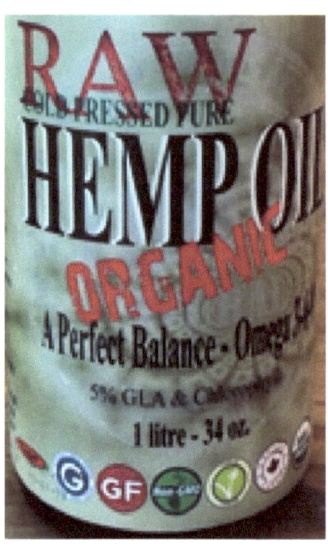

Raw shelled hemp seed and hemp seed oil are one of nature's perfect foods. Raw hemp (hemp seed or hemp seed powder or hemp seed oil, pictured above) provides a broad range of health benefits including, but not limited to: increased and sustained energy, weight loss, rapid recovery from disease or injury, lowered cholesterol and blood pressure, reduced inflammation, improved circulation, improved immune system as well as it acts as a natural blood sugar control. Another benefit in consuming hemp seed including hemp seed oil is improved digestion.

Modern science shows that hemp contains all the essential amino acids and essential fatty acids necessary for optimal human health, along with a rare protein known as globule edestins that is very similar to the globulin found in human blood plasma.

NOTE: Oils should be pressed with a minimum of heat because the higher the temperature of the oil, the faster it is destroyed by light, oxygen and other chemical reactions. The shape and properties of Fatty acid molecules can change and thereby lowering their nutritional and biological value. Therefore, always look for organic cold pressed oil when choosing your brand.

Hemp seed oil is also a rich source of both Omega 6 (LA) and Omega 3 (LNA) essential fatty acids in balanced proportions. This means that conditions caused by deficiencies in either can be treated by one oil, hemp.

The functions of Omega 3 or LNA include: smooth skin; improved stamina; healing; increased vitality; increases the feeling of calmness; enhances immune functions; reduces pain and swelling associated with arthritis; can reverse PMS; increases brain development in children and can treat bacterial infections.

The functions of Omega 6 or LA include: production of energy; increased vitality , mental state and oxygen transfer; assists in a speedy recovery from fatigue; assists with the production of important secretions; builds immunity; prevents allergies and the functioning of heart tissue.

It has been reported that a lot of information about hemp has been systematically removed from written texts since the 1930's and is now difficult to find.

Hemp Seed Oil Medicinal Salad Dressing Recipe

The following recipe can be adjusted to suit your taste. It can be varied by substituting red wine vinegar or lemon juice for the apple cider vinegar. It is your choice how much or whether to add garlic and turmeric powder. I recommend that you do try the following recipe as it provides a very powerful immune boosting ability.

Oil to vinegar in a 3 to 1 ratio (3: 1) meaning for each three tablespoons of hemp seed oil, add one tablespoon of vinegar or lemon juice.

3 Tbsp. Hemp seed oil

1 Tbsp. Apple cider vinegar (ACV)

2-3 cloves garlic crushed

¼ - ½ tsp. turmeric powder

Crushed black peppercorn

Himalayan salt to taste

Whisk together Hemp oil and ACV and add the balance of the ingredients and whisk thoroughly. Adjust the Himalayan salt and fresh ground pepper to your taste. Toss with your favorite greens and chill before serving for best tasting salad ever.

Noteworthy

EXTRACTUM CANNABIS
Extract of Cannabis
Ext. Cannab.—Extractum Cannabis indicæ P.I.

Prepare an extract by percolating 1000 Gm. of cannabis, in moderately coarse powder, using alcohol as the menstruum. Macerate the drug during forty-eight hours and then percolate it at a moderate rate until the drug is exhausted. Evaporate the percolate to a pilular consistence at a temperature not exceeding 70° C., and mix the mass thoroughly.

AVERAGE DOSE—Metric, 0.015 Gm.—Apothecaries, ¼ grain.

From USP 1936 page 155

The above is from the United States Pharmacopeia 1936 – partial information on cannabis before its removal.

In the 18th century Persian medical text *Makhzan-al-Adwiya*, written by M.Husain Khan, cannabis was described in its various preparations as an intoxicant, stimulant and sedative, but also the following:

"The leaves make a good snuff for deterging the brain; the juice of the leaves applied to the head as a wash, removes dandruff [sic] and vermin; drops of the juice thrown into the ear allay pain and destroy worms or insects. It checks diarrhea, is useful in gonorrhea, restrains seminal secretions, and is diuretic. The bark has a similar effect. The powder is recommended as an external application to fresh wounds and sores, and for causing granulations; a poultice of the boiled root and leaves for discussing inflammations, and cure of erysipelas, and for allaying neuralgic pains."

Conclusion

This book has provided you with an introduction to the raw cannabinoids or cannabinoid acids along with the terpenes found in the cannabis plant. When phytocannabinoids (those found in the cannabis plant) are activated, either by heating or through oxidization, aging (degradation) or prolonged UV light, they lose the chemical molecule or the A and are then said to be neutral.

Although the majority of relatively current scientific studies on cannabis focused only on THC, the scientific community is beginning to study the powerful and synergistic benefits of this as a whole; the sum is worth more than its parts.

As patients become more aware of the amazing qualities of the cannabis plant and of the complexities in the compounds found in the various cannabis strains, they will become more discerning when choosing the medicine that is right for them. This in turn will lead to a market lead by consumers rather than one controlled by profit mongers, with little concern for the patient. In other words, it is within our constitutional right to demand "patients before profits"!

ABOUT THE AUTHOR

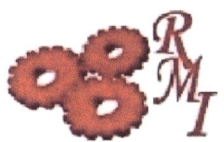

Ryder Management Inc.
"putting you in gear"

Ryder Management Inc. (Rydermgt) is a Canadian Controlled Private Corporation (CCPC) based in London, ON Canada. As an "umbrella" organization, it brings together a group of authors whom are professionals in their respective fields and are writing with the primary goal of providing books that educate, comfort and offer assurance that natural remedies do exist and are an effective and safe way to enhance health.

The contributing author of our first book "*A Cancer Cure? The Amazing Health and Beauty Benefits of Turmeric*" was diagnosed with cancer and adamantly refused conventional cancer treatment used in Canada. She then began a quest for an alternative method of treatment that included online research, interviews and placing calls to India. It was fate to have been subsequently put in touch with "Rick Simpson".

www.ingramcontent.com/pod-product-compliance
Lightning Source LLC
Chambersburg PA
CBHW050857290526
45792CB00002B/634